Beautifully Made!

Celebrating Womanhood
(Book 2)
Fourth Edition

Edited by
Julie Hiramine

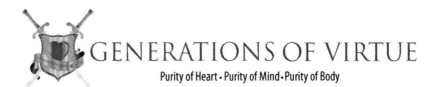
GENERATIONS OF VIRTUE

Purity of Heart · Purity of Mind · Purity of Body

Contributors:

Julie Hiramine	Beth Lockhart	Megan Briggs
Mary Whitlock	Annie Anderson	Kelsey Roberts
Sara Raley	Chris McCausland	Katherine Lockhart

All contributions were made as a free-will gift to Generations of Virtue

Beautifully Made! Celebrating Womanhood
Copyright © 2003 by Generations of Virtue
Fourth Edition © 2011 by Generations of Virtue

Published by: Generations of Virtue
                  P.O. Box 1353
                  Monument, CO 80132
                  www.generationsofvirtue.org

Scripture quotations are taken from The Holy Bible, New King James Version Copyright © 1982 by Thomas Nelson, Inc.

Printed in the United States of America
ISBN: 978-0-9766143-1-9

Table of Contents

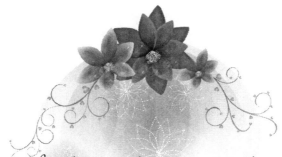

For you formed my inward parts; You covered me in my mother's womb.

I will praise You, for I am fearfully and wonderfully made; Marvelous are Your works, and that my soul knows very well.

My frame was not hidden from You, When I was made in secret, and skillfully wrought in the lowest parts of the earth.

Your eyes saw my substance, being yet unformed. And in Your book they all were written, The days fashioned for me, When as yet there were none of them.

—Psalm 139:13-16

Preface

Beautifully Made! is a three-book series designed to guide daughters and their moms through the passage from girlhood to womanhood. You hold in your hands the second book in the series, Celebrating Womanhood. This book is for young ladies who have started their periods. It is a guidebook for girls who are experiencing the newfound spiritual and physical changes associated with becoming a woman.

If you have not started your period yet, you'll want to read the first book in the Beautifully Made! series, which is called Approaching Womanhood. This book is full of practical information about body changes, the biology behind the menstrual cycle, and growing up. It also includes words of encouragement and guidance for girls and their mothers to make the transition from girlhood to womanhood a positive experience.

Book 3 in the series is called Wisdom from a Woman and is written to the moms, aunts, guardians, or grandmothers who are going to be going through the books with their girls. This third book gives mom an encouraging message as she prepares to share with her daughter about the beauty of God's design for a woman's body. Full of practical tips and stories from other moms, Wisdom from a Woman provides support and advice in a timely manner.

Celebration

Psalm 1:3a[1]

He shall be like a tree planted by the rivers of water that brings forth its fruit in its season.

First of all, congratulations! You are now officially a woman! You always were female, but now you're able to experience what gives us the ability to create life. While you may be embarrassed and think "What is going on, and why do I have to read this book?" this time is actually a fabulous one, full of newness and excitement. Let's talk about why. God designed you to be a "tree of life"—literally. A fabulous description of all the science and biology behind your period is presented in the first book of this series, <u>Approaching Womanhood</u>, but in this part I really want to get across how important this time is spiritually. God is pleased. I know another thing you may be thinking: You'd rather no one know about what is going on with you or your body.

1. All scripture is taken from the New King James Version (NKJV) of the Bible unless otherwise noted.

And for awhile, no one really needs to know—except those people around you whom you can trust and ask for advice: your mom, sister, grandmother, or teacher, that's up to you.

God has given you the power to make life. Your body is actually changing and developing into a place that can house and grow life, kind of like a greenhouse would with plants. He doesn't give us this gift lightly. He expects us to respect life and treasure it the way He does. He values life so much that He sent His son to die so that we could keep on living. He says that our bodies are a temple, and we are to treat them that way.

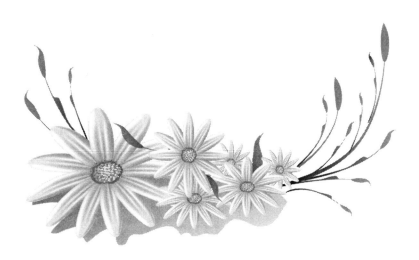

So be excited and encouraged. This is a good time; it is a time to celebrate. Don't be surprised when your mom, sister, grandmother, aunt, or friend wants to celebrate with you. You should rejoice in the goodness and awesome wonder of God, that He has made you who you are, and you are a woman. Let's pray this prayer:

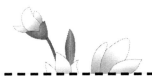

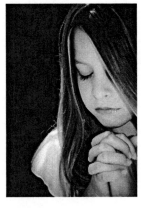

"Dear Lord, thank you for making me a woman. Thank you that you've given me the ability to make life. 'I praise you because I am fearfully and wonderfully made.' (Psalm 139:14) I want to always bring glory to You with my body. Help me to respect and treasure life the way You do. Teach me what it means to be a woman, the way You designed me to be. Help me to understand Your purpose for my life and how being a woman fits into Your perfect plan."

Signed:_____

Date:_____

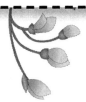

Choices

After you start your period, you need to know the different options that you have for taking care of yourself. There are many choices when you go to the store to buy products. In this section I talk about two different options.

Pads

One of the most common products that women use is the pad. Pads are made of soft cotton and fit in your panties. They have a plastic bottom to prevent leaks and are also sticky on the bottom so they will stay where you put them. Pads come in many shapes and sizes that you can buy according to how heavy or light your flow is when you are on your period.

It is usually a good idea to find out which type of pad feels the most comfortable. It might be a good idea to ask your mom which kind she uses, although you might like something different. To insert a pad, remove the paper backing and stick it on your panties a little toward the front. To dispose of the pad, wrap it in the wrapper that comes with it or in toilet paper and throw it in

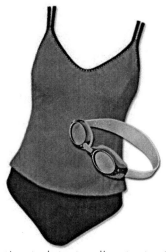

the trash. Never flush a pad down the toilet. It will get stuck and cause the toilet to overflow, which can be embarrassing besides causing a lot of problems. In most toilet stalls of public restrooms there is a trash can of some kind just for the purpose of throwing away these pads. Sometimes pads are a disadvantage, like when you want to go swimming. It is not a good idea to go swimming with one on. It would soak up a lot of water and feel uncomfortable. This method is also unsanitary to use in water because everything on the pad could leak into the water.

Tampons

A tampon is the other most popular product to use while on your period. It is made of absorbent cotton and fits inside your vagina. The tampon has a string attached at one end so you can pull it out when you are finished with it. There are many choices with tampons. The best choice for you most likely will be the junior or slim fit. Be sure to never use super absorbency tampons at this stage in your development. These junior tampons also come in different

varieties. The junior tampon with a plastic applicator is the easiest to use. Bigger tampons will be more difficult to use in the beginning. You can start with the small size and when you are more comfortable with using tampons, you can upgrade to a larger size if needed.

To insert a tampon for the first time, you need to already have blood flowing. If you try to insert a tampon while you are dry, it will probably hurt and not work well. Another very important reason to wait is that having a tampon in when you don't need one could be dangerous. If you read the directions on a box of tampons you will see a section talking about TSS (toxic shock syndrome), an illness that develops very rarely but is a serious concern. This illness is caused by bacteria building up in your vagina when you are using the same tampon for too long a time or using a tampon with too high an absorbency for your blood flow. Symptoms of toxic shock syndrome are as follows: fever over 102 degrees, faintness or dizziness, diarrhea, nausea or vomiting, and a sunburn-like rash that is painless.

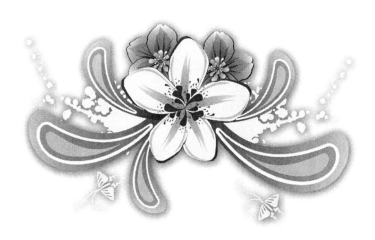

CAUTION

You should always let your mom or another responsible adult know that you are using tampons in case you start to feel the symptoms of TSS. Tampons are a good option if you want to go swimming while on your period. Unlike a pad that would leak in the water, tampons are fine in water because they are inside you where water cannot reach.

Using a tampon

Some women find a tampon too difficult to use the first time. This does not have to be the case with you. Don't be nervous if it doesn't work the first time you use one. Wait and try again another time. When using a tampon for the first time, it might be a good idea to lie down on your back. One of the most important things to do before you try to put a tampon in is to relax. Using a tampon is new to you and may seem a little strange. If you relax, it will go much easier because your muscles will not be tense, thus making it easier to insert. Remove the paper wrapping and notice there is an applicator with the cotton tampon inside.

There is also a string hanging out of the bottom of the tampon; this is to remove the tampon when you are finished using it. Insert the tampon into your vagina and push upwards and back towards your spine at the same time. When the top part of the applicator is mostly into your vagina, push the bottom half of the applicator into the top. Next, remove the applicator and the tampon will stay inside you with the string hanging out.

You may leave a tampon in for four to six hours but not longer. It is very important that you change your tampon regularly. If you start to leak sooner than this, change to a fresh tampon. Some women wear a panty liner (a very thin pad) to protect their panties if they do leak a little bit.

Make sure that when you are finished you remove the last tampon. It is very easy to forget that the tampon is in because it will not leak to remind you. To dispose of the tampon applicator, wrap it in toilet paper and put it in the trash.

Some tampons say they are flushable. You may flush your tampon if the box says so, unless you are in a place that has plumbing problems or a sign saying not to flush feminine products or if your home uses a septic system. If this is the case or if the tampon is not flushable, then wrap it in toilet paper and put it in the trash. It is a good idea to make sure your pad or tampon is covered up in the trash can. Please be considerate of the next person who uses the restroom. It is not pleasant to see pads or tampons in the trash after they have been used.

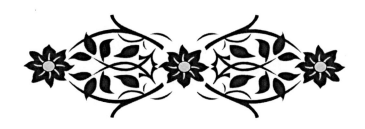

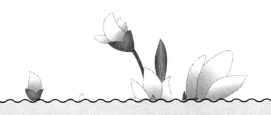

The first time that I ever used a tampon was my freshman year in high school. And let me tell you, for me, the timing could not have been worse. I was on my way to Hawaii (literally en route), and I started. So, when we arrived in Hawaii I was crushed. Maui was full of beaches and pools and I couldn't enjoy any of them because I could not use a tampon. I decided to take a shower as everyone else was heading down to the pool. I remembered that God cares about every aspect of our lives—even using tampons! So, as weird as it may be, I asked Him to help me. As soon as I got out of the shower and dried myself off, I went straight for the tampon box. I was able to use one without any pain or discomfort. Praise God for His answer to prayer!

Kelsey

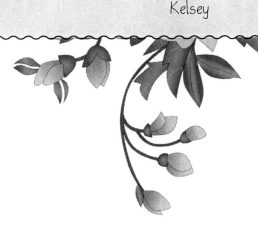

How to Insert a Tampon

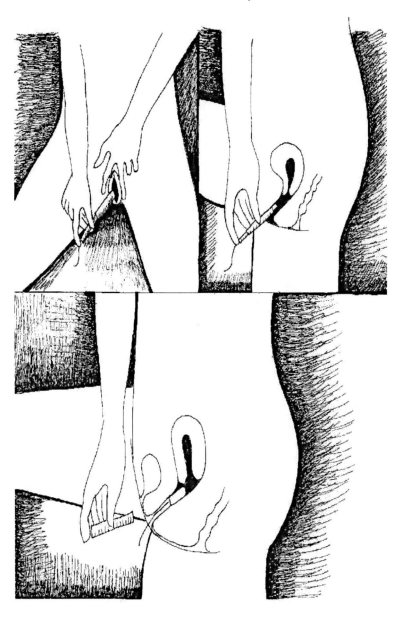

Keeping Track of Your Cycle

It's a good idea to keep track of your cycle by using a chart like the one on page 27. Most girls do not have a consistent cycle the first few years after they start their periods, but charting your cycle will help you keep track of when you will probably start next and if your blood flow follows a pattern. It's helpful to know approximately when you will have your next period so you can plan accordingly and bring products with you wherever you go.

The charts on the following pages include a calendar year of recording your period. On our example chart on page 27 this girl started her period February 12th. To chart this, she would find the month February on the left-hand side of the chart and then slide her finger over to the 12th (the numbers are located directly under the words "Menstrual Record Chart). In this box, where February and the number 12 meet up, is where she made a mark.

You have three options for marks: an "X" represents a normal blood flow. This is the amount of blood that is common for you whenever you are on your period. An "O" represents light blood flow. This means your blood flow is slightly lighter or less than normal. Finally, if you were to color in the whole box, that mark represents a heavy blood flow.

In a typical menstrual cycle, you will probably experience all three kinds of blood flows. For most girls, the first day of their cycle is pretty normal, the second day might be a little heavier, the middle days are pretty normal, and then the last day is light.

Another symbol we used in the example chart is an "S". This represents spotting, where you may bleed a very little bit, but not enough to be considered a light blood flow. This spotting typically happens right before you start your cycle.

Finally, we also give you a symbol to track when you experience PMS. There is more information about PMS later in this booklet, but for right now just know that "P" represents PMS.

Don't worry if your menstrual cycle does not follow this pattern; everyone is different and no two women have the same cycle.

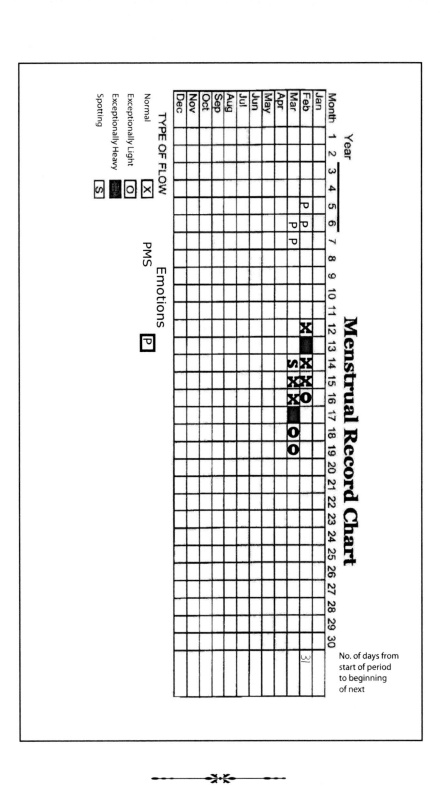

Menstrual Record Chart

Year ________

Month	1	2	3	4	5	6	7	8	9	10	11	12	13	14	15	16	17	18	19	20	21	22	23	24	25	26	27	28	29	30	No. of days from start of period to beginning of next
Jan																															
Feb					P	P						X	■	X	X	O															31
Mar						P	P							S	X	X	■	O	O												
Apr																															
May																															
Jun																															
Jul																															
Aug																															
Sep																															
Oct																															
Nov																															
Dec																															

TYPE OF FLOW

Normal	X
Exceptionally Light	O
Exceptionally Heavy	■
Spotting	S

Emotions

PMS	P

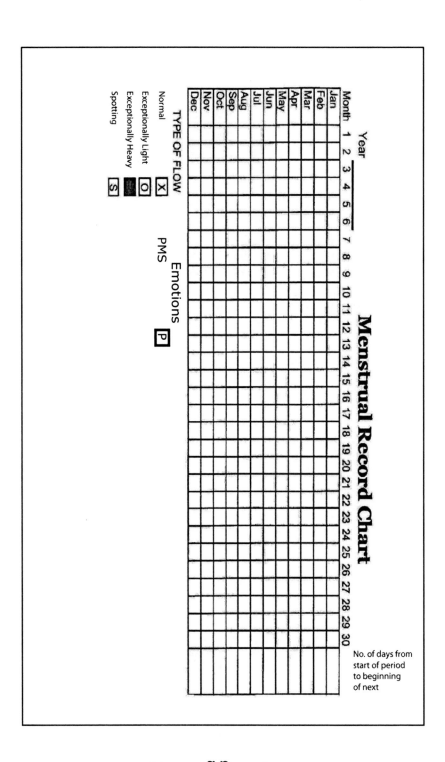

Menstrual Record Chart

Month	1	2	3	4	5	6	7	8	9	10	11	12	13	14	15	16	17	18	19	20	21	22	23	24	25	26	27	28	29	30
Jan																														
Feb																														
Mar																														
Apr																														
May																														
Jun																														
Jul																														
Aug																														
Sep																														
Oct																														
Nov																														
Dec																														

Year

No. of days from start of period to beginning of next

TYPE OF FLOW

Normal ☒
Exceptionally Light ◻
Exceptionally Heavy ◼
Spotting ⬛

Emotions

PMS ℗

29

PMS

2 Corinthians 1:5
For as the sufferings of Christ abound in us, so our consolation also abounds through Christ.

Have you ever heard someone say "I'm PMSing"—maybe a sister, or your mom? PMS, premenstrual syndrome, is something you may have already heard about or are just starting to hear about. PMS is what can happen about 7-10 days before you start your period each month. It's a good thing to at least be aware of PMS so that when and if it happens, you'll know what to expect. Some of the symptoms you may experience are:

- Depression
- Mood swings
- Breakouts/more pimples
- Aches and pains (in your back, muscles, breasts)
- Irritability

- Headaches
- Loss of control
- Insomnia
- Cravings (like chocolate!)
- Bloating (water retention)

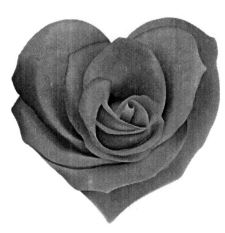

Learn to recognize how you feel during the month. Because having your period is only one part of your cycle, the rest of the month may be changing and feel different also. If you begin to experience any of the symptoms in the list above, rest assured, you are normal, and almost every woman experiences some sort of PMS symptom before starting her period. When these things do happen, it's good to recognize it. Don't let your feelings outrun you. Don't get too upset at things that you know aren't a big deal. Here's a funny example of someone who was experiencing PMS: One of my friends told me how, when she was in school, she was going through the lunch line and while she normally had 1% milk to drink, that day they were out of it. She said she almost started crying right there in the lunch line!

I've had plenty of experiences like that one. I already have a tendency to be dramatic, so when that time of the month comes, things can get a little crazy. My mom has said a couple of times, "Are you about to start your period? You've been grouchy and upset all week!"

You may be going through your day like normal and someone may say something, or maybe your clothes aren't fitting as well, or maybe your brother is ten minutes late picking you up—all of these things, while PMSing, can cause tears, heartache, and downright pain.

When these things happen, we need to take a deep breath and realize what our bodies are going through. Once you learn what the routine is for your body, you can plan things around that. Take a day to just chill out, don't make plans that Saturday afternoon if you know you're going to feel a little under the weather; give yourself time to rest.

Another part of this booklet helps you understand some of the natural remedies for dealing with cramps and PMS symptoms. I encourage you to read that section and try out those remedies. The first step is knowing what's going on. Like I said, learn to recognize what your body goes through, what the routine is. If it helps you to chart it out and write it down, then do it. Certainly don't feel alone—we all know what PMS is like.

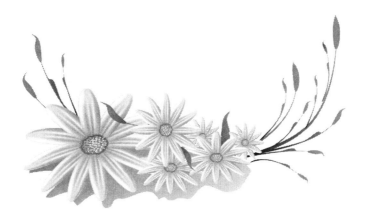

What Happens When You Mature Younger Than Your Friends?

Song of Solomon 6:9a
My dove, my perfect one, Is the only one.

As you move into womanhood, you may notice that your cycle is different than the cycles of other girls. Have no fear, I was the same way. I started my period in fifth grade, at age ten. I began showing signs of puberty around age nine, so it wasn't too surprising when my period came so early. For the first few years, I struggled with starting my period at a younger age than my friends, and I also had some problems with cramps. For young women who start menstruating at an early age (before junior high school), adjusting can sometimes be difficult. I recommend having your mom call your teacher and explain your situation. This will greatly reduce your stress and really put you at ease knowing that someone can help you when your mom is not around. This way, your teacher

can be sensitive about bathroom trips, cramping, etc. I recommend buying a small, purse-like container in which to put feminine products so that you can discreetly take tampons and/or pads to the restroom. If you are using pads, try finding thin ones that will work and keep them in your back pocket, preferably in some sort of container.

Now, let me stress that over the past year or so, my cycles have regulated and my cramps have greatly decreased. I believe that this has come about by changing the way I view my period. God has blessed us with the amazing capacity to produce human life. The Bible says, "Sing to the LORD, for he has done excellent things!" (Isaiah 12:5) I urge you to pray this prayer whenever you are feeling stressed or frustrated about your period.

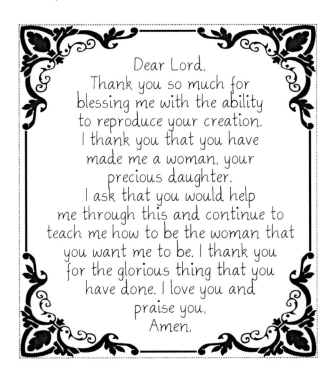

Dear Lord,
Thank you so much for blessing me with the ability to reproduce your creation. I thank you that you have made me a woman, your precious daughter. I ask that you would help me through this and continue to teach me how to be the woman that you want me to be. I thank you for the glorious thing that you have done. I love you and praise you, Amen.

Help in Time of Need

Hebrews 4:16
Let us therefore come boldly to the throne of grace, that we may obtain mercy and find grace to help in time of need.

There are some symptoms you may experience when your period starts. Some girls experience things like back aches, headaches, nausea, and cramps. If you develop cramps or back pain, there are ways to obtain relief. Make sure that you are full; cramps on an empty stomach are worse. Take hot baths, and stay in as long as you are comfortable. Heating pads have been a lifesaver. An electric heating pad with a high, medium, and low setting is a great investment. Exercise is also very important. Cardiovascular workouts will help regulate and decrease cramping.

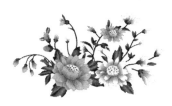

My best advice: Work out at least three times a week; make sure some of this is cardiovascular. Healthy bodies handle periods best. A natural supplement we have found to work well if you are having problems with your period or cramping is Evening Primrose Oil or Total EFA Flaxseed Oil, which has Evening Primrose Oil in it. This product can be found at a health foods store. The best way to take this is in its oil form. If you find you don't like the taste of the oil, you can disguise it in flavored yogurt. Our experience has been that this supplement makes periods lighter.

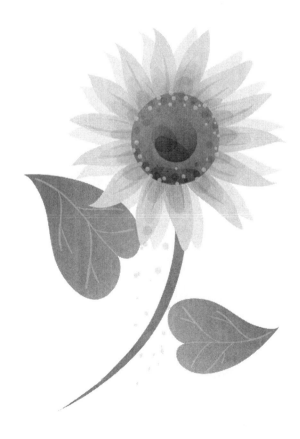

Period Tips

You may have a lot of questions now that you've started your period. Here are some answers to some of the most frequently asked questions girls ask about their periods.

If you don't use tampons

You might be invited to do something like swimming while you are on your period. If you don't use tampons, this may present a conflict for you. But don't worry: everyone has to turn down an invitation from time to time on account of their period. Sometimes you don't feel quite yourself, and it's better to stay home. If this happens to you, explain the situation to your parents. They will understand. You may have your mom or dad write you a note if you need to be excused from something like a school or camp activity.

Also, if the situation arises, you may need to explain to the person who invited you why you cannot come. It's ok to feel a little embarrassed, but know that any woman is going to understand.

Travel
When you travel, be sure to bring products with you. Even if you don't think you will start while you are on your trip, make it a habit to bring at least a few products with you. Especially the first few years you have your period, sometimes your cycle can be a inconsistent. You may not be expecting to start sometimes. For this reason, travel with products just in case. If you carry a purse or backpack with you regularly, put products in a discreet zippered pocket or in some kind of pouch. There may even be times when you may not need the products yourself but can help out a friend who forgot to bring them.

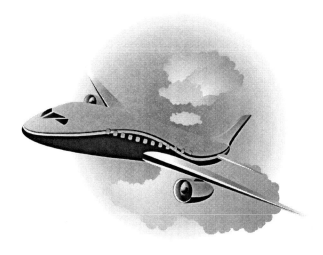

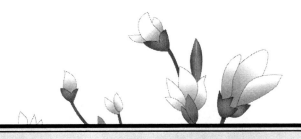

One time I was traveling in Asia when I started my period. I was just about to board a plane for a 15-hour flight and realized I didn't have any products on me! I had started unexpectedly and I left my products in the bag I checked. I raced around the airport terminal and finally found a convenience type of store. The only problem was the lady was closing the shop right then! I frantically tried to explain to her that I needed to buy products. But she only spoke Chinese and didn't understand anything I was saying. She motioned for me to wait and brought back a young guy who looked to be about 18. I was so embarrassed, but I had no choice. Obviously this young man spoke English and so I explained to him why I was there, delaying the closing of their shop. The poor guy was just as embarrassed as I was. It was a hard lesson to learn, but I now travel with products on me wherever or whenever I go.

-Julie

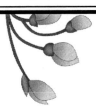

Public Restrooms
Some public restrooms do not have trashcans in every stall. If you are in a restroom like this and need to dispose of a feminine product, simply wrap the pad or tampon in some toilet paper and take it with you when you leave the stall. Throw it away in the trashcan provided for paper towels when washing your hands.

Wearing White
Unfortunately, sometimes you can leak while you are on your period. You may have seen another woman who has leaked onto her clothes. To avoid this, wear dark bottoms (pants, shorts, capris, or skirts) while you are on your period. This doesn't mean that you can never wear white, but it may take you some time at first to know when you need to change products and how to avoid leaking on your clothing.

Leaking
If you find yourself in public and you realize you've leaked on your clothing, don't panic. If you have a sweater or something you can tie around your waist and cover your rear end, start with that. See if you can borrow a friend's sweater if you don't have your own. Next, go to the restroom and change your products. If the stain is visible from the outside of your clothing, you can try getting it out with water and paper towel. Take some wet paper towel into a bathroom stall and try blotting the stain out. When you get home, you will probably need to continue treating the stain.

Conclusion

1 Chronicles 29:13
Now therefore, our God, we thank thee,
and praise thy glorious name.

Now that you have started your period, it is very important to be a good steward of your body. The dictionary defines the word steward as "a person who manages another's property". You see, God has given you this body and this life. It is not your sole property. What this means is that you need to take care of your body as if it belongs to someone else: namely, God.

How do you take care of your body? First of all, eating good foods and getting plenty of rest are good places to start. You can also make sure to exercise on a regular basis and keep up good hygiene. Finally, there are a lot of harmful things you can do to your body. You want to avoid things like smoking and tattoos, especially at this age. Your body is still growing and developing; it is in a sensitive state. Be careful to do everything you can to build a strong, healthy body.

This stage of your life is so full of potential and possibility. It's a great time to seek God's will for your life. You never know what God will have you do in the future, but you can prepare now by making daily prayer and Bible study a part of your life. You can also honor God by taking care of the body He has given you.

Lastly, congratulations once again! May God bless you and keep you as you mature into the woman He has called you to be.

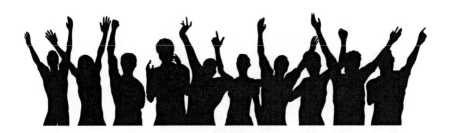

A Word About Generations of Virtue

The mission of Generations of Virtue is to equip parents, churches, schools and organizations to empower the next generation to be pure in our world today. Generations of Virtue isn't just a ministry   it's a movement to turn the tide of culture. Starting in 2003, GOV was founded by Julie Hiramine out of a realization that parents are facing a world that is intent on trampling their children's purity of heart, mind and body. Parents need to be prepared to train their kids to stand against this force from the enemy as they answer God's call on their lives. The questions are everywhere:

- How do we live lives of purity and integrity?
- Why is God's love story so much better than what the world has to offer?
- How can this generation see the Living God and His incredible plan for their lives?

Generations of Virtue is passionate about providing the latest, cutting-edge resources, dynamic teaching sessions and engaging tools that groups, churches, parents, teens and families can use to stand pure before God in heart, mind and body.

For upcoming events, practical resources, and to join the movement of raising up a holy generation, visit our website:

www.generationsofvirtue.org

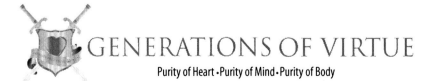

GENERATIONS OF VIRTUE

Purity of Heart · Purity of Mind · Purity of Body

If you enjoyed this book, please check out the other books in the <u>Beautifully Made!</u> series:

Approaching Womanhood

Book 1 in the <u>Beautifully Made!</u> series.

Designed for mother-daughter discussion and bonding time. Help your daughter through this potentially stressful experience while she anticipates her first period. This book is designed to encourage your daughter as it discusses issues all developing girls face and wonder about: her changing body, her first period, her body image, how she can be prepared if her period starts unexpectedly, and, most importantly, her worth in God's eyes and her role in God's Kingdom. Recommended for girls ages 8-12.

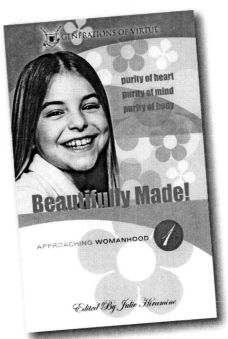

www.generationsofvirtue.org
Purity of Heart, Purity of Mind, Purity of Body

Wisdom From A Woman

Book 3 in the <u>Beautifully Made!</u> series.

Are you anxious about your daughter starting her period? Generations of Virtue has compiled a wonderful resource for mothers to lovingly guide their daughters into womanhood. This book contains ideas on how to celebrate with your daughter, an informative section on the biology behind women's bodies, how and when to tell your daughter about her period, and some of the surprises associated with a developing daughter (for instance, mood swings). This Biblically-focused book can help every mother explain some of the intricacies of womanhood to her precious girl.

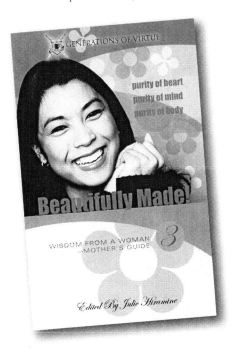

This book is for mothers of preteen girls.
Find this three-book series at www.generationsofvirtue.org

Available On Audio CD!

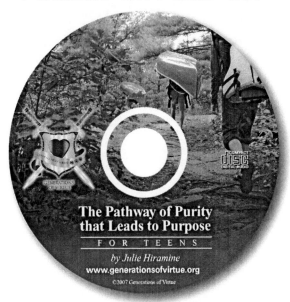

Using the 5 senses of seeing, feeling, tasting, hearing, and smelling, **Julie Hiramine** will not be your science instructor, but edifying you in order to stay pure. In today's world, there is a flood of inappropriate imagery and explicit content that besieges us everywhere we turn. God's call on this generation is to step up into His higher standard and seek His face in the midst of all that wants to pull us off course. Teens need to learn how to navigate through the maze the world is currently lost in with their eyes on Jesus as their guide. Teens will receive practical guidance on how to meet the many challenges that surround them in the areas of dating versus courtship, media discernment, and developing a deeper relationship with the Lord in this captivating presentation.
Recommended for teens and parents.

www.generationsofvirtue.org
Purity of Heart, Purity of Mind, Purity of Body

CPSIA information can be obtained at www.ICGtesting.com
Printed in the USA
BVOW02s1618160414

350604BV00005B/7/P

9 780976 614319